Linda Has Lupus
Copyright © 2016 by Sheronda S. Hayes-Burt
Edited by S. S. Rowell

Acknowledgement
The American College of Rheumatology, Google,
Bing, Pinterest Images.
Cover & Inside illustrations by Ms. Tileya Hardmon.

Printed in United States of America

This book is dedicated to my grandchildren, Brooklyn, Madison, Kendall, & Kandis.

Linda is a seven-year-old girl who has Lupus. (Lupus is a disease that attacks the body).

The children at school tease Linda because of the butterfly rashes that appear on her face, mainly across her nose because of the Lupus.

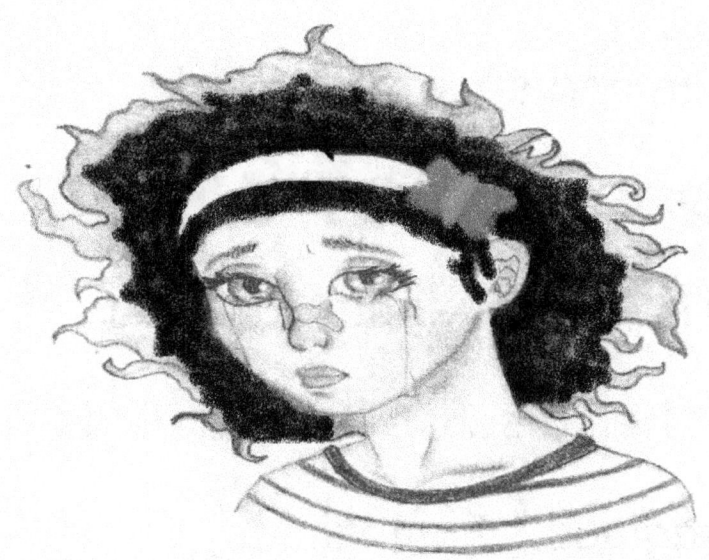

One day, Linda was playing with her friends, Madison, Brooklyn, and Kandis, when two boys came near them and shouted, "Linda has a disease, run." Brooklyn, one of Linda's friends shouted," You can't get her disease because it is not contagious." Sometimes, people can be so mean to others that are different than they are, or have an illness that they do not understand.

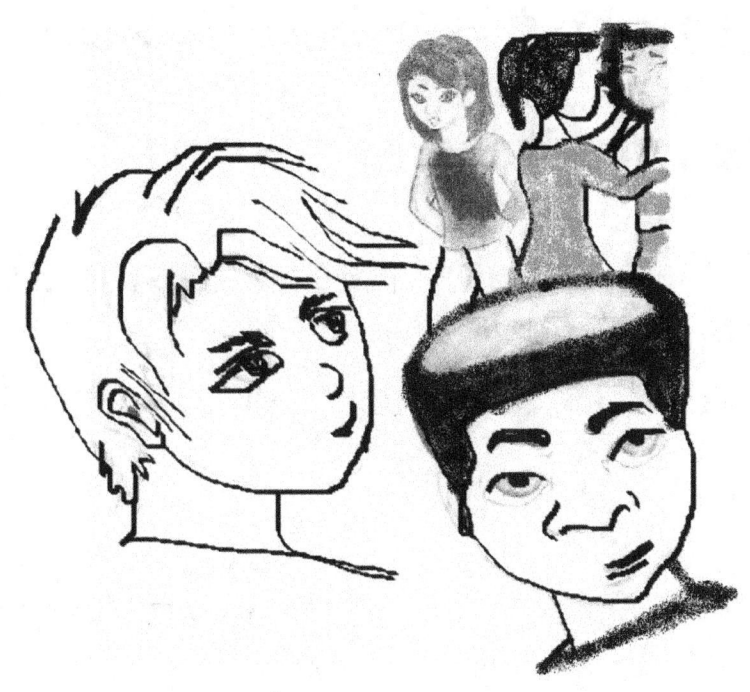

Linda can't go outside like most children when the sun is shining too bright because it can irritate her Lupus. (Sensitivity to the sun's UV rays is another symptom of Lupus).

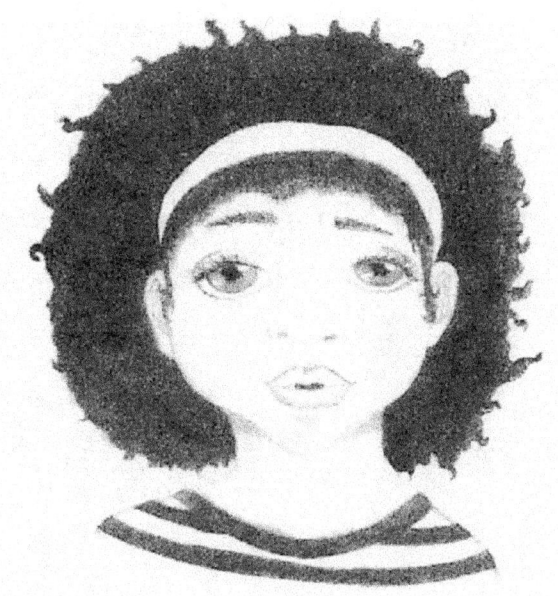

Whenever Linda go outside on a sunny day, she must wear a huge hat, or use an umbrella, and sunglasses.

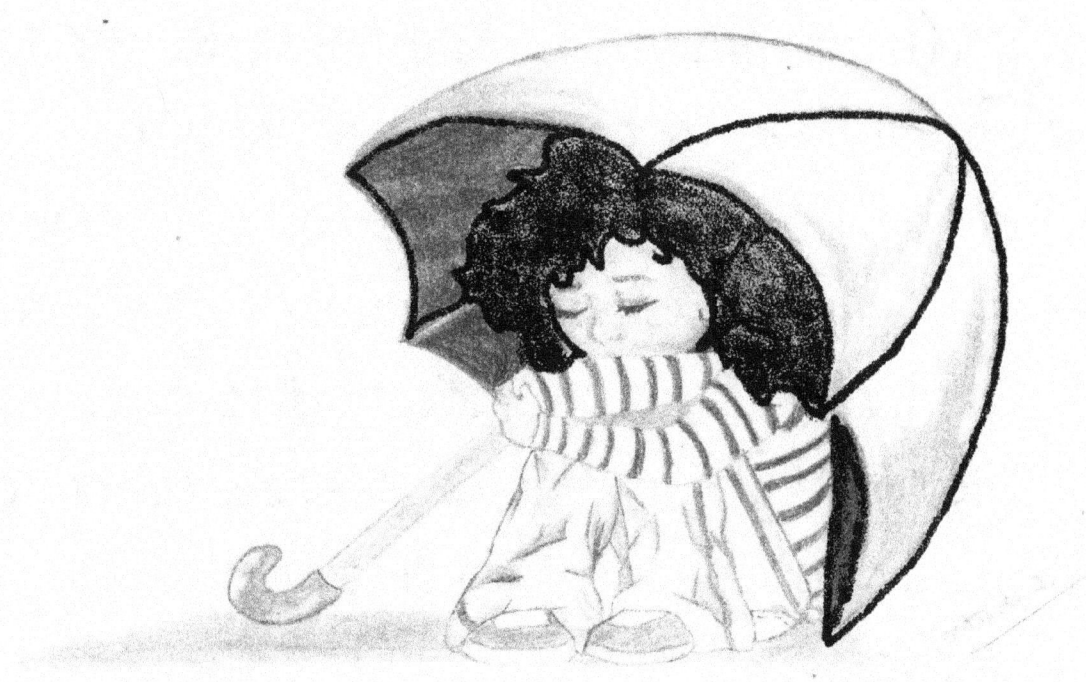

Linda goes to the doctor who is a Rheumatologist. (A Rheumatologist specializes in treating people with arthritis, which is a painful inflammation that also causes stiffness of the joints). During this visit, Linda had to get her blood drawn and urine tested to make sure that everything was working properly.

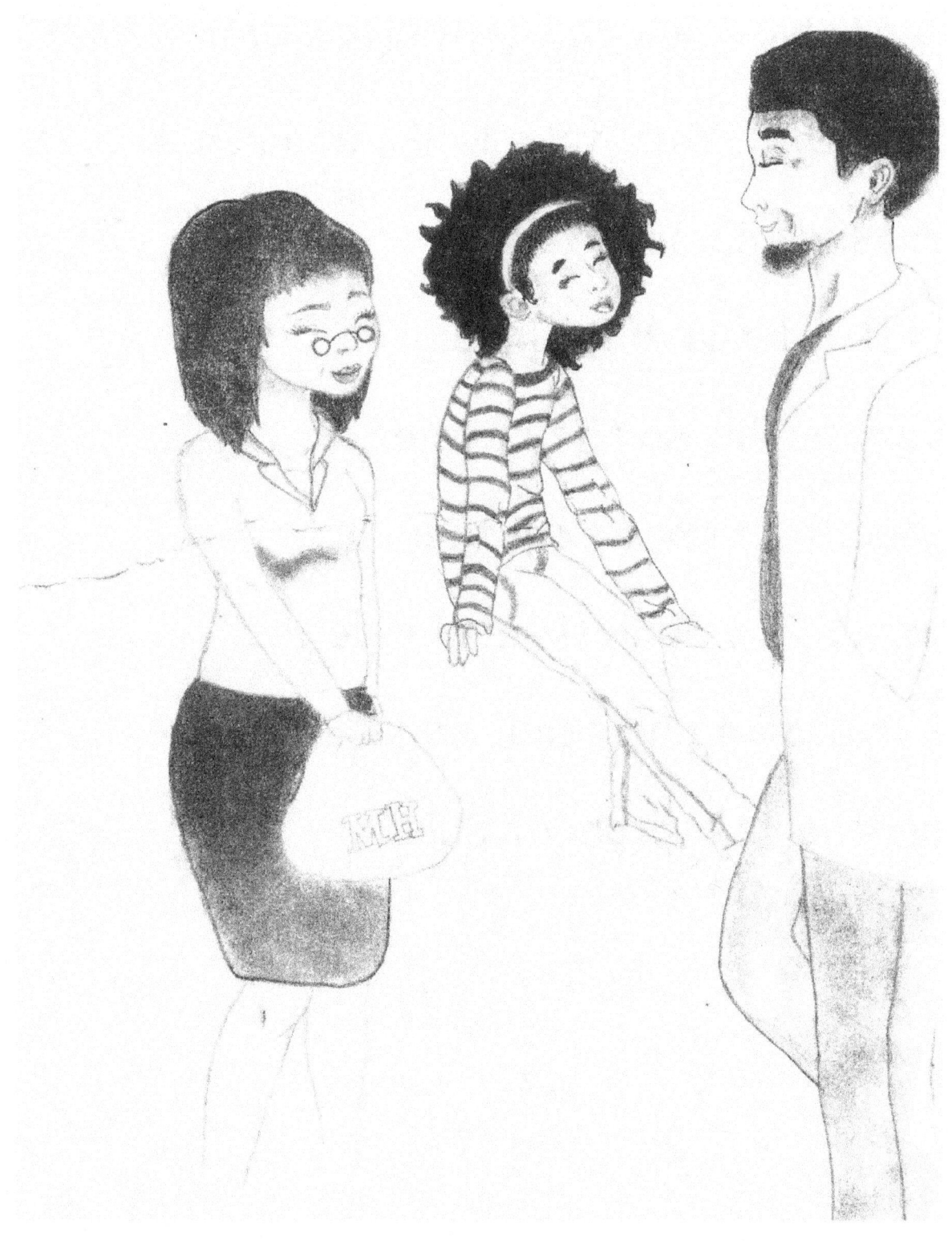

Linda loves to play with her dog Scrappy. They take walks and run around the house while having loads of fun, but Linda gets tired very easily, so the both of them usually lie down together and watch TV. Sometimes, Linda just likes to sit and read. (Fatigue is another symptom of Lupus).

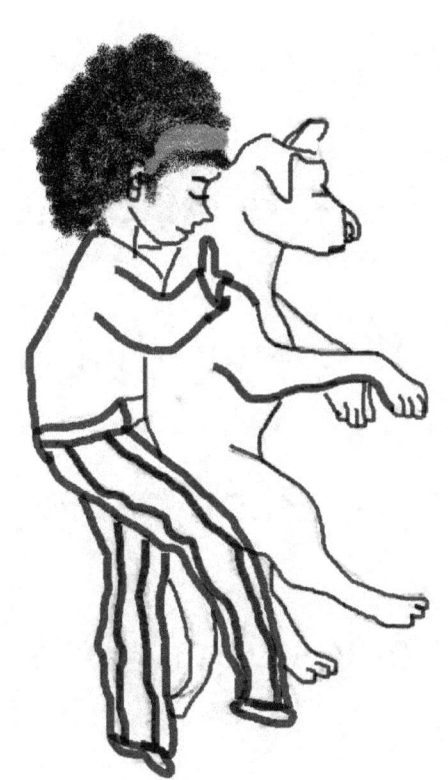

On many hot, summer days when she can't go outside to play, Linda enjoys staring out of the window at the beautiful butterflies that dance around the flower garden. After daydreaming, Linda enjoys reading upside down. Reading helps Linda concentrate on stories about beautiful things, people, and places instead of her pain from Lupus.

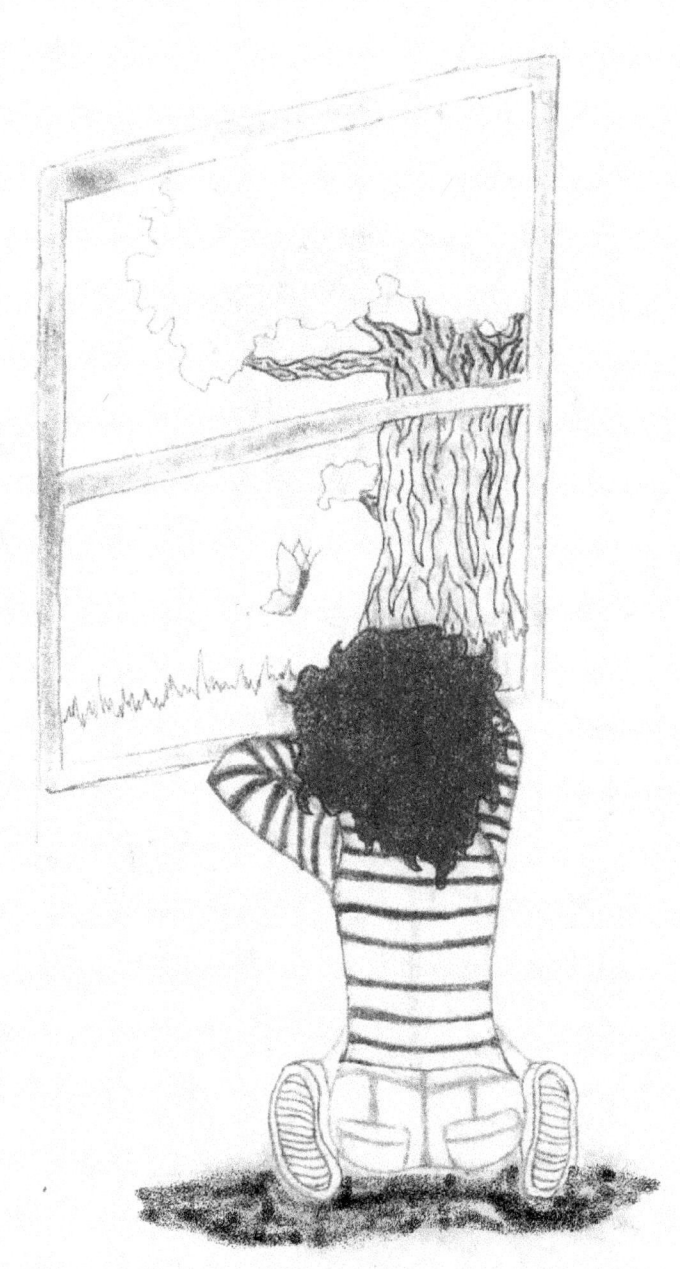

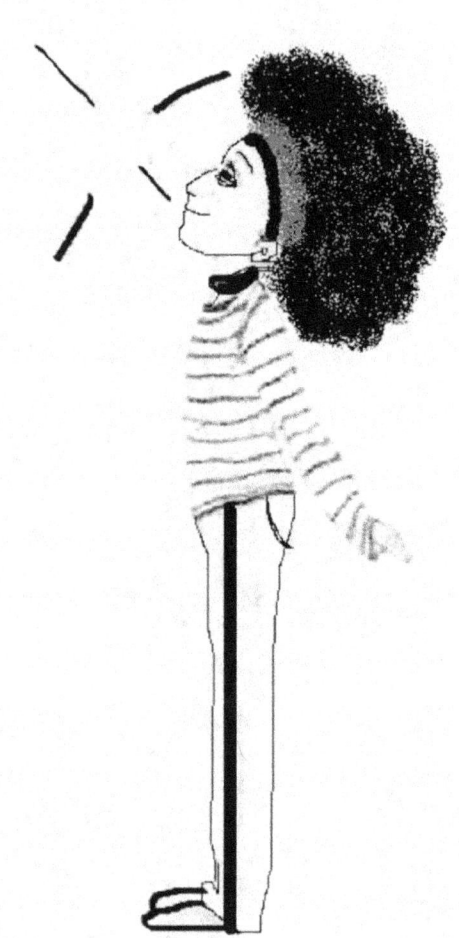

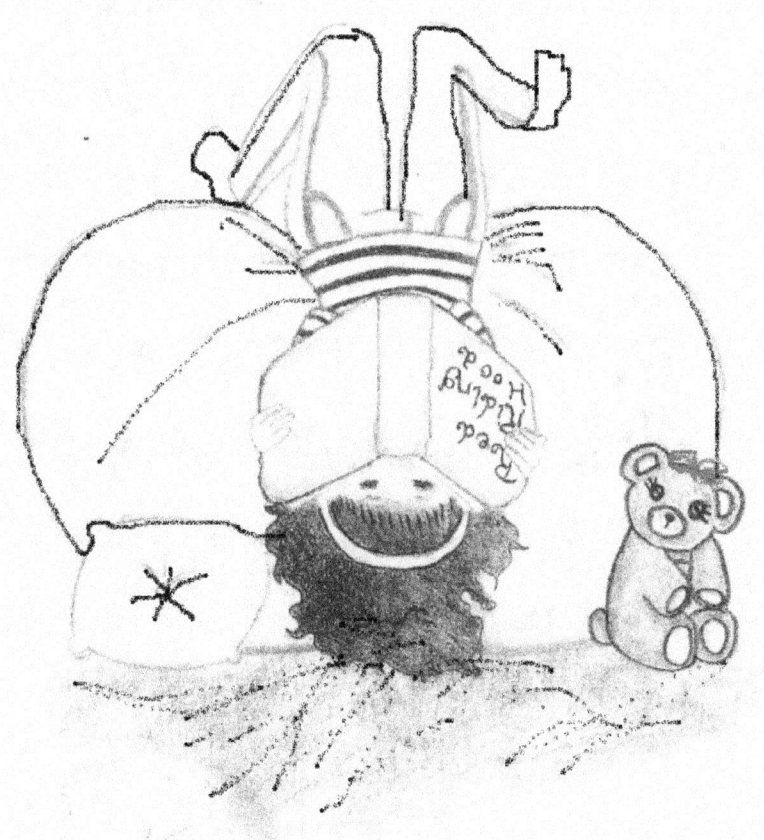

Linda says her prayers every night before bedtime, praying that the next day will be a better one than the last one. Linda will have Lupus for the rest of her life, or at least until a cure is found. Although Linda has her family and friends to help her get through the pain and agony of this disease, she still has her moments of frustration, but she has her faith to hold on to and that makes a world of difference.

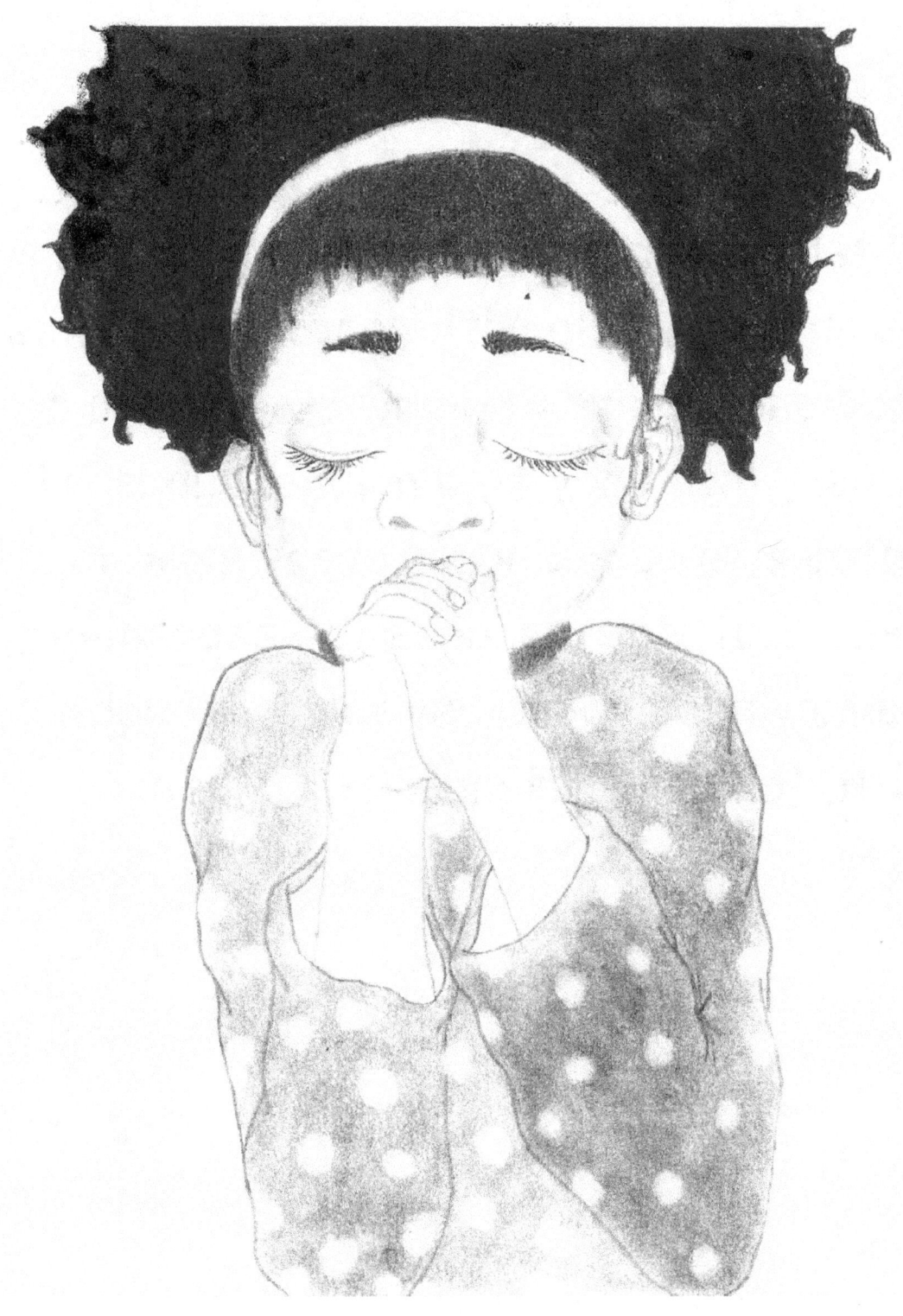

Butterflies are free and able to explore the outside world with no worries, unlike Linda and others who share her form of Lupus. Until they find a cure, Lupus will continue to rule Linda's every move in life.......but, she manages to keep smiling and moving forward any way, through faith, family, & friends!

Systemic Lupus Erythematosus (Juvenile)

A study about Lupus in children was updated in July 2013 by Lori Tucker, MD, British Columbia Children's Hospital, and Sandra Watcher, RN, BSN, Children's Hospital Los Angeles, and reviewed by the American College of Rheumatology Committee on Communications and Marketing. The following is a list of fast facts offered in this study: ***Lupus is a chronic disease, with flares and remissions. ***Lupus is not contagious and it cannot be prevented. ***Lupus can affect many different areas of the body. ***Treatment is different for each child; each child is unique, as is each treatment plan. ***Lupus and several medications used for lupus suppress the immune system. *** Work with your rheumatology team to learn about lupus and find the best treatment plan to control it. ***Becoming more involved in your care will help as you grow with this illness to make choices and transition into adulthood. - See more at: http://www.rheumatology.org/I-Am-A/Patient-Caregiver/DiseasesConditions/Systemic-Lupus-Erythematosus-Juvenile#sthash.pS5IvDN2.dpuf

Write Your Thoughts Here

Write Your Thoughts Here

Write Your Thoughts Here

A cure has not yet been found for Lupus, nor has anyone discovered what causes it, but, the search for a cure and more answers is an ongoing process....so, come join the fight for a cure!!!!!

www.ingramcontent.com/pod-product-compliance
Lightning Source LLC
Chambersburg PA
CBHW081544280526
45788CB00010B/3350